CINNAMON

MARIAN KIM

CONTENTS

1

PROPERTIES

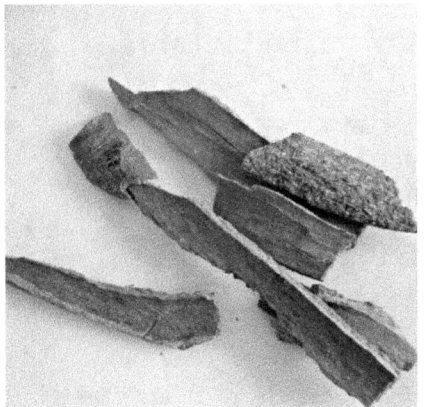

Scientific name: Cinnamomum zeylanicum

Other names: Canelle, cassia, dalchini

Nutrients: Cinnamon has a high fiber content.

Properties

Anti-inflammatory properties

Anti-oxidant properties

Anti-aging properties

Antiseptic (antibacterial, antiviral, antifungal) properties

Anti-cancer properties

Immune system boosting properties

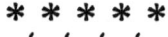

2

USES

Diabetes

Cinnamon is used for diabetes treatment. A German study proved that cinnamon improves blood sugar control in people with type 2 diabetes by reducing their blood glucose level. This can be achieved by taking just 1/2 teaspoon of cinnamon each day. Cinnamon can also prevent diabetes. This was shown by a study done by *The Center for Applied Health Sciences* in which participants who were given 250mg of water soluble cinnamon each day were found to have an increase in the antioxidants associated with lowering blood glucose levels.

Intestinal spasms relief

The German Commission E which is a governmental advisory board approves the use of cinnamon for the management of mild gastrointestinal spasms.

Anorexia treatment

The German Commission E approves the use of cinnamon for the management of anorexia since it stimulates the appetite.

Indigestion treatment

The German Commission E approves the use of cinnamon for the management of indigestion. It is also used to manage flatulent dyspepsia and dyspepsia with nausea. Cinnamon is also used to soothe upset stomachs.

Flatulence relief

Cinnamon is a carminative which is used to relieve flatulence (gas). It is also used to manage colic.

Prevent nausea

Cinnamon is used to prevent and relieve nausea including that caused by morning sickness.

Treat diarrhea

Cinnamon is used to treat infantile diarrhea because it has mild astringent properties.

Relieve heart burn

Cinnamon is used to relieve heart burn.

Acne treatment

Cinnamon is used for acne treatment because it has antibacterial, anti-inflammatory and anti-oxidant properties. When the powder is used to form a treatment paste, it also has an exfoliating effect since it helps remove the dead surface skin cells.

Urinary tract infection (UTI) treatment

Cinnamon is used to treat UTIs (urine infections). It has been shown to suppress Escherichia coli which is the bacteria which causes most UTIs.

Menopausal symptoms relief

Cinnamon is used to manage menopausal symptoms.

Menstrual problems management

Cinnamon is used for menstrual problems since it can help regulate the menstrual cycle. It contains tannins which have astringent properties and are useful for reducing bleeding from heavy periods. Cinnamon is also used for painful menstrual periods.

Nosebleed management

Cinnamon contains tannins which have astringent properties and are useful for reducing bleeding from nosebleeds.

Lowering high cholesterol

Cinnamon is used for lowering cholesterol levels. A study revealed that cinnamon can lower the levels of the total cholesterol, the LDL (bad) cholesterol and triglycerides. This can also be achieved by taking just one quarter of a teaspoon of cinnamon per day.

Heart disease prevention

Cinnamon is used to prevent heart disease. Cinnamon prevents heart disease by lowering cholesterol levels and blood sugar levels and by being rich in anti-oxidants called polyphenols.

Weight loss

Cinnamon is used for weight loss. Cinnamon helps regulate blood glucose levels by reducing the insulin surges that occur after meals and contribute to food cravings. It is therefore doubly effective for diabetics trying to lose weight.

High blood pressure treatment

Cinnamon is used for lowering high blood pressure.

Colds and coughs management

Cinnamon is used to reduce the symptoms of colds and coughs especially when it is combined with ginger.

Stress management

Cinnamon is used for stress management since it has a tranquilizing effect that is also useful for anxiety reduction.

Erectile dysfunction treatment

Cinnamon is used to manage erectile dysfunction (ED).

Joint conditions

Cinnamon is used to manage joint conditions.

Chest pain relief

Cinnamon is used to relieve chest pain.

Bedwetting

Cinnamon is used for bedwetting.

Antiseptic

Cinnamon is used as an antiseptic because it has antibacterial, antiviral and antifungal properties. Cinnamon contains compounds which can kill bacteria like Salmonella, Escheria coli (E. coli) and Staphylococcus aureus. It also suppresses the fungi Candida that causes thrush.

Insect repellent

It is an effective insect repellent.

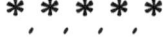

3

SAFETY PRECAUTIONS

1. Persons using medications for lowering blood sugar levels should use cinnamon with caution since it can also lower blood sugar levels.

2. Since it can interfere with blood sugar levels, persons scheduled to have surgery should stop using it at least 2 weeks before the operation date.

3. Persons with liver disease should use cinnamon with caution since it contains a chemical which can cause or worsen liver disease.

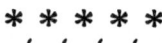

4

DRUG INTERACTIONS

1. Cinnamon can interact with antidiabetes medications and lower blood sugar levels.

2. Cinnamon can interact with medications that can harm the liver and cause liver damage especially in people with existing liver disease. Examples of medications with the potential to harm the liver include acetaminophen (Tylenol), carbamazepine (Tegretol), isoniazid (INH), methotrexate (Rheumatrex), fluconazole (Diflucan), itraconazole (Sporanox), phenytoin (Dilantin) and simvastatin (Zocor).

* * * * *

5

COOKING TIPS

Flavor: Sweet woodsy

Goes well with: Pumpkin, rice, breads, milk shakes, orange desserts

Can be substituted with: Nutmeg, allspice

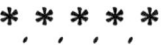

6

HERBAL RECIPES

Cinnamon Tea

Equipment

Kettle

Tea cup

***

Ingredients

1 teaspoon of cinnamon powder

1 cup of boiling water

Honey to taste (optional)

***

Instructions

1. Put the cinnamon in a tea cup, add the boiling water and let it steep while covered for 10 -15 minutes.

2. Add honey (if using) to suit your taste before drinking.

*****

Cinnamon Syrup

Equipment

Saucepan

Jar with airtight lid

***

Ingredients

1 quart (1000 ml) filtered water

1 cup cinnamon

1 cup honey

***

Instructions

1. Place the water and cinnamon in a saucepan and bring to a boil.

2. Reduce the heat and let it simmer while it is partially covered until the volume is reduced to half the original volume.

3. Strain the mixture through a sieve or cheesecloth to remove the cinnamon.

4. Measure 1 pint (500 mls) of the liquid and add the honey.

5. Cook for a few minutes as you stir it so that it thickens.

6. Store the syrup in an airtight container in the fridge for up to 2 months.

*****

Cinnamon Butter

Equipment

Large glass bowl

Electric mixer or stick blender or wire whisk

Molds such as ice cube trays (optional)

***

Ingredients

½ cup butter

2 tablespoons cinnamon powder

***

Instructions

1. Place the butter in a warm place so that it can soften.

2. Put butter and cinnamon in a large glass bowl and blend well until thoroughly mixed.

3. Refrigerate until it hardens. You can refrigerate it in molds or ice cube trays to give it a special shape.

*****

Cinnamon Acne Paste

Equipment

Glass bowl

***

Ingredients

1 teaspoon lemon juice

½ teaspoon cinnamon powder

***

Instructions

1. Mix the cinnamon powder with enough lemon juice to make a smooth paste.

2. To use, apply the cinnamon paste to the acne pimples and wash it off with warm water after 20 minutes.

***

Tips

1. Mix the cinnamon powder with honey to make an overnight acne treatment paste that can be rinsed off in the morning.

*****

Cinnamon Infused Oil

Equipment

Double boiler

Large glass bowl

Sieve and cheesecloth

Sterilized dark jars

***

Ingredients

16 fl oz. (500 ml) vegetable oil like sweet almond or sunflower oil

8 oz. (250 grams) cinnamon

***

Instructions

1. Place the cinnamon and oil in the glass bowl ensuring that the oil covers the spice. Simmer them in a double boiler for one hour at a temperature of around 120 degrees Fahrenheit (49 degrees Celsius). Do not let the mixture boil. You can repeat this step several times after letting the oils cool to create more concentrated spice infused oils.

2. Strain the mixture through the sieve and cheesecloth into a clean, dark jar ensuring you squeeze out as much oil as you can from the cheesecloth.

3. Label your jars and store your spice infused oils in a cool dark place or in the refrigerator and use them within 3 months.

*****

Cinnamon Salve

Equipment

Double boiler

Large glass bowl

Sterilized dark jars or tins

***

Ingredients

8 oz. (250 ml or 1 cup) cinnamon infused vegetable oil (see previous recipe)

1 oz. (30 grams) beeswax

50 drops (2.5 ml or ½ teaspoon) essential oils like lavender essential oil (optional natural fragrance)

***

Instructions

1. Place the beeswax and cinnamon infused oil in the glass bowl and melt them in a double boiler.

2. Once melted remove from the heat source, allow to cool and add the essential oils (if using).

3. Pour the melted oils into the storage jars or tins and allow to cool completely.

4. Store the salves in a cool dark place.

***

Tip

If you want softer salves you can use less beeswax – for example ¾ oz of beeswax for 1 cup of vegetable oils.

*****

Cinnamon Lip Balm

Equipment

Double boiler

Large glass bowl

Lip balm tubes or small jars or tins

***

Ingredients

3 tablespoons cinnamon infused vegetable oil (see recipe above)

1 tablespoon grated beeswax

1 tablespoon shea butter

***

Instructions

1. Place the beeswax, shea butter and cinnamon infused oil in the glass bowl and melt them in a double boiler.

2. Once melted remove from the heat source and pour into lip balm tubes and allow to cool completely.

*****

Cinnamon Tincture

Equipment

Glass jar with tight fitting lid

Dark tincture bottles

Cheesecloth

Labels

***

Ingredients

7 oz (200 gm) of cinnamon

30 oz (1 liter) of 80-100 proof vodka

***

Instructions

1. Fill 1/3 of the glass jar with the cinnamon.

2. Add the vodka to completely fill the jar to the top.

3. Seal the jar and label it with the date of preparation and name of spice used.

4. Store the glass jar in a dark place for 6 weeks ensuring that you shake them weekly.

5. After 6 weeks strain out the cinnamon with a cheesecloth and pour the tincture into dark tincture bottles.

6. Label the tincture bottles with the date and name of herb used.

7. Store your herbal tinctures away from light and heat.

***

Tips

1. You can leave the herbs in the alcohol for up to 6 months if you want to create very strong tinctures.

###

ABOUT THE AUTHOR

Marian Kim is an experienced alternative medicine practitioner.

OTHER BOOKS BY THE AUTHOR

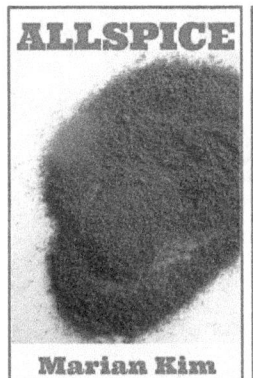
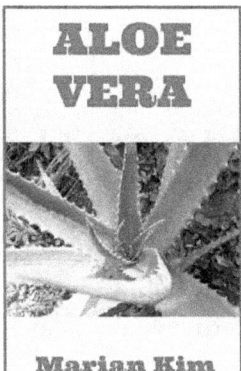
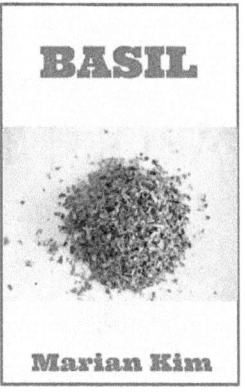

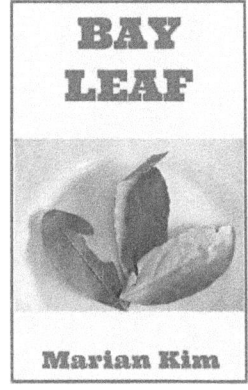
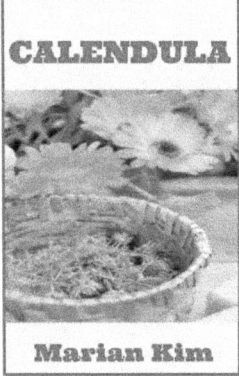
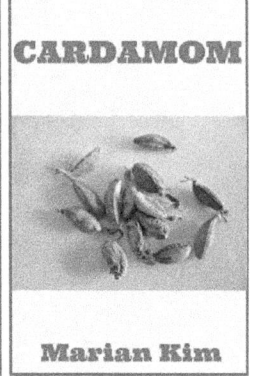

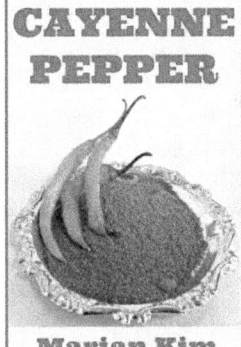

CAYENNE PEPPER

Marian Kim

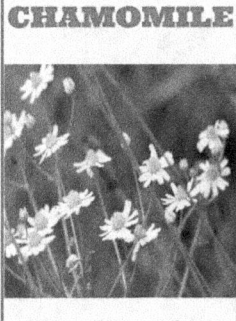

CHAMOMILE

Marian Kim

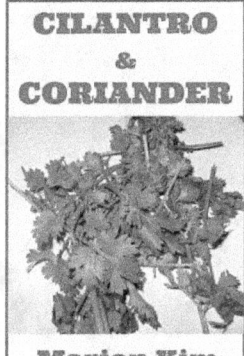

CILANTRO & CORIANDER

Marian Kim

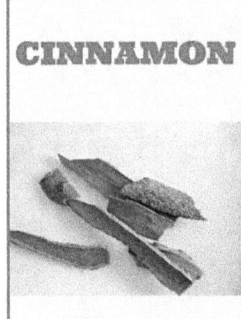

CINNAMON

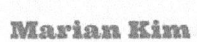

Marian Kim

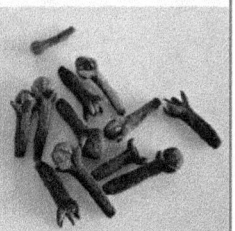

CLOVES

Marian Kim

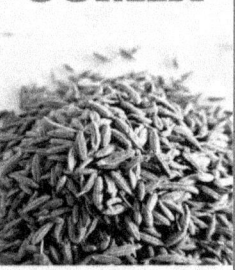

CUMIN

Marian Kim

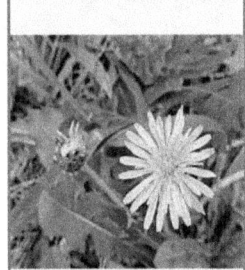

DANDELION

Marian Kim

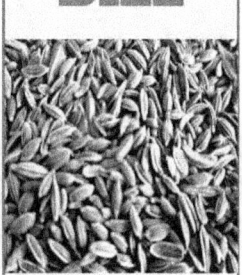

DILL

Marian Kim

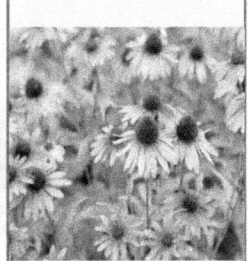

ECHINACEA

Marian Kim

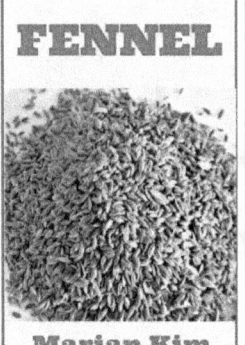

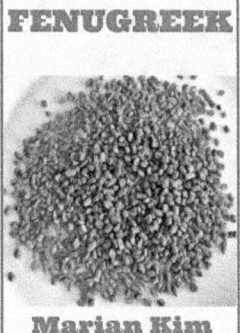

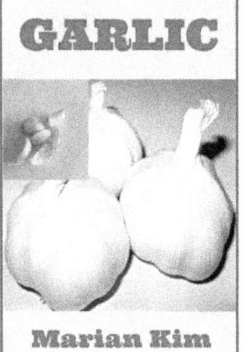

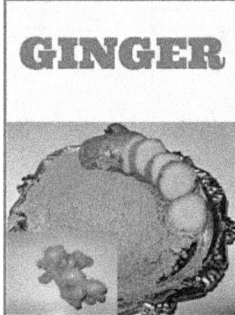

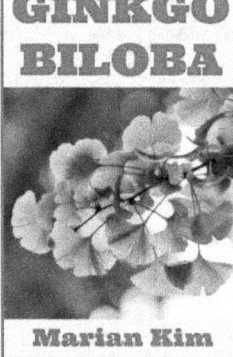

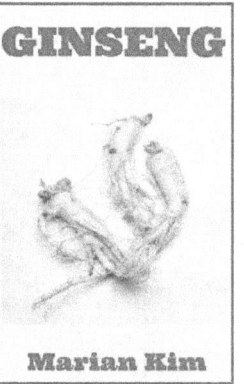

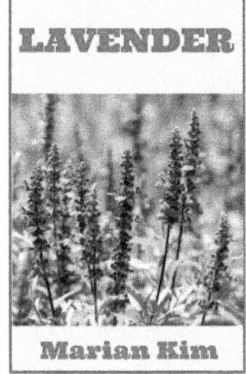

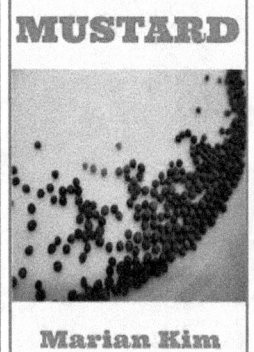

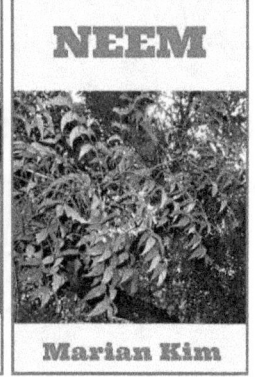

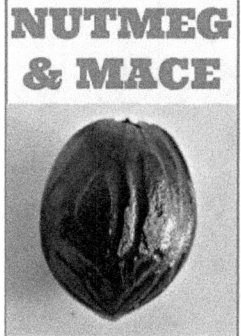

NUTMEG & MACE

Marian Kim

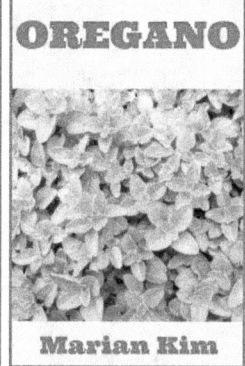

OREGANO

Marian Kim

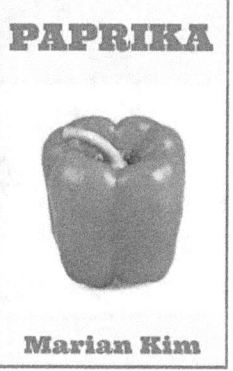

PAPRIKA

Marian Kim

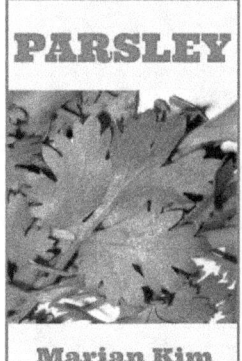

PARSLEY

Marian Kim

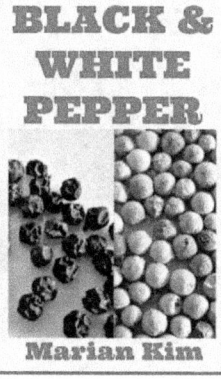

BLACK & WHITE PEPPER

Marian Kim

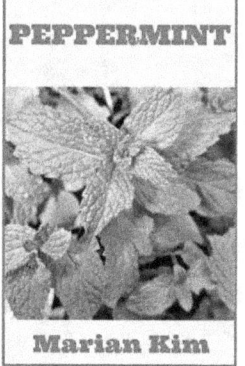

PEPPERMINT

Marian Kim

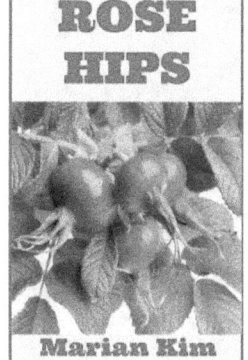

ROSE HIPS

Marian Kim

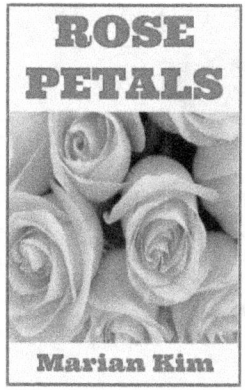

ROSE PETALS

Marian Kim

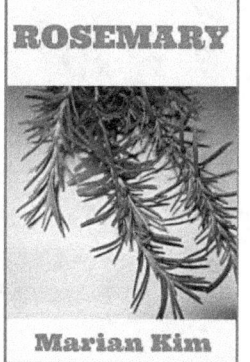

ROSEMARY

Marian Kim

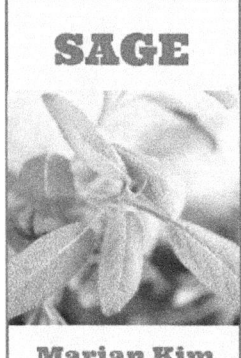

SAGE

Marian Kim

ST. JOHN'S WORT

Marian Kim

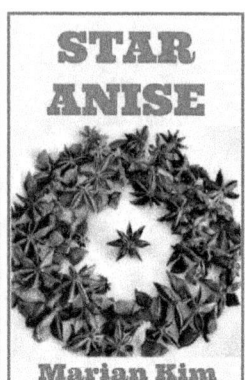

STAR ANISE

Marian Kim

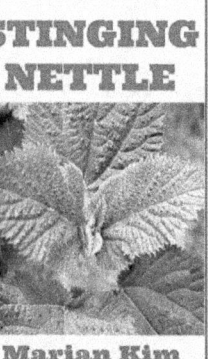

STINGING NETTLE

Marian Kim

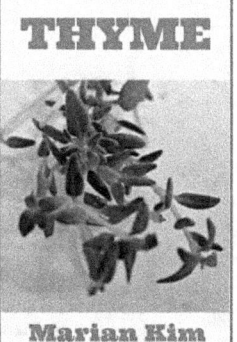

THYME

Marian Kim

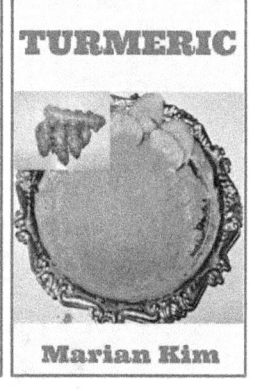

TURMERIC

Marian Kim

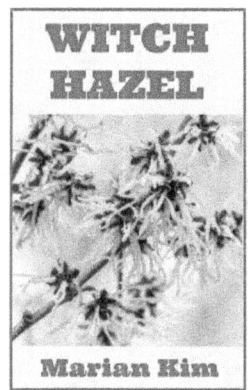

WITCH HAZEL

Marian Kim

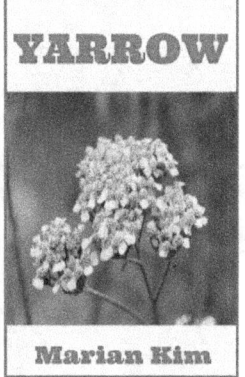

YARROW

Marian Kim

*****